Copyrigh

MW00895486

Library of Congress Cataloging-in-Publication Data

Ladouceur, Debby, 1953-
        Handbook   for   Happiness/Debby Ladouceur
        ISBN 978-1-304-25589-1 (paperback)

ACKNOWLEDGEMENTS

Debby has lived in the Canadian Rocky Mountains with her husband and two sons for the past 25 years. Her family is surrounded by wilderness and the beauty of the natural world, the mountains, valleys, and streams that form the upper Fraser River watershed.

In that time, some of the skills & tools she has acquired and uses to facilitate health include nutritional & wellness counseling, herbal medicines, Iridology & Reflexology. She has assisted many people "in achieving their best in health, spirit, mind and heart. Finding and simplifying the successful regime unique to each person is the goal. Compliance and choice are always in the hands of the client. I have no doubt that health and happiness are possible for everyone."

I gratefully acknowledge the assistance and editorial contributions of Claris Cowan and David Salayka. I sincerely thank my family and friends who have provided unwavering support in many forms including ideas, editing, discussions, etc. My sons and husband and two big dogs have and continue to be my greatest teachers.

INTRODUCTION:

Congratulations! You have chosen to consider happiness in your life, or in the life of someone you know. I know there are many self help books out in the world. My goal is to simplify and break down into steps how to create and expand happiness in your life. To those who have read and researched ways to better understand themselves and their lives; this book is a concise reminder of the importance of the simple steps that initiate leaps in your life. To those who have not been inspired by other books, or find themselves so embedded in life that happiness has been left by the wayside, this book will be a wonderful guide for taking the first steps. Reading this book will remind you of how deserving of happiness you are and how rewarding your life can become.

If a society is successful, its people are happy. Most people have been so shaped and managed by culture, religion, governments, TV and society in general that they are no longer in touch with their true selves. I have come to understand that every action, every thought, every emotion are choices we make moment by moment, day by day, even year by year. I believe we must understand choice, and realize that society itself has orchestrated and in many ways created our roles for us: depressed, rebellious, irritable, timid, victim, poor, angry, sick, etc. Important to keep in mind is not to blame or create victimhood within yourself because of your particular situation, but recognize and become aware that it is your choice to take a step in the direction of change in your own life. It is time now to re-create two of the missing puzzle pieces: curiosity and common sense.

The world around us is ever-evolving; all species of plants and animals adapt or die. It doesn't matter that life spans are longer and science is awesome–it appears to me that humans are de-evolving. We have moved so far away from being part of the miracle of life on a spectacular and vibrant planet that we've become stuck in epidemics of depression, disease, violence and every form of disrespect possible to living beings.

So isn't it time to wake up, become calm and make choices to change your life? Step up to the plate and, whatever else you do, don't underestimate 'happiness'.

The role you play is not who you are, it's what you have settled for in a society that has lost its way. The brilliance of being happy is that it takes all aspects of your life, job, relationships, parenting, politics, etc., to the next level. So the change I speak of is **how** you live the life you have chosen.

Our human body is made up of trillions of individual cells, grouped into organs and communities to work collectively for our personal common good. I am going to give you very simple steps to take with mind, body, heart and soul to improve every aspect of your being and your life, measureable by you in whatever goals you may set. Be your own experiment and follow any or all of the following steps for only seven days and you will attain measureable, positive results.

We have all been bamboozled; brain washed, or robbed of our own sense of self by a society that has gone wild with exploitation, industry, technology, devalued food and an attitude about money that is totally out of proportion to its true value. I can guarantee you this–no matter your degree of happiness or lack thereof at this moment, you can raise your place on the happiness scale. When you invite a small measure of happiness into your life, expanding on what you already have, you begin a gradual filling up that will surprise you each day, each week, until you find yourself grateful, happy and moving in a direction of personal success and wonderment. How you feel, what you think, what you eat, what you choose to say, do, give, and take are very small choices you make all day long. Most people have become observers in their own lives rather than participants. This is what you will change. A smile can change your destiny. Remember, it takes 26 muscles to smile and 62 muscles to frown.

Many people I have communicated with over the past 25 years in regard to wellness are so keen to hear this, enthused to imagine wellness for them, and they walk out the door with a new perspective. Within hours, days, or months, however, many return to the state they started in. We simply have to choose; that is where the first step lies on any journey. If you are a parent, teach your children as early as they are able to listen, to incorporate these steps into their young lives. The best of positive habits will begin to flourish and the results will surprise your entire family, their teachers, and their friends. It is where it all must begin.

I realize that each person has their own unique life situation and I do not in any way mean to diminish or naively overlook the fact that many are in despair. Many are in relationships, jobs, lives that may appear so troubled that a discussion of happiness sounds absurd. If you are a person in despair or a person who sees no hope for happiness, the most important thing I would ask of you, is this: In a safe moment take a step back, see one single thing you might change, one tiny shift that might move you forward.

Throughout any scenario in your life the **truth** is all that matters. Not your version or my version of truth. Real Truth exists; there are laws of nature at work within each of us, gut feelings of right and wrong, a sense of beauty, of feeling safe. I am astounded to notice that happiness, joy and love have been placed so high on their pedestals that, to many, they seem forever out of reach. Define what "happy" is to you. Find a picture of a moment in your life that was full of promise and happy to recall; as I have done with the photo on the cover of my book. Speak of it, if only to yourself, so your brain hears the words, gets the message and steps up to the plate to help you find a way. It can be as simple as waking up and deciding today is going to be a good day. It is a sense inside that all is well. No matter how great the obstacles, you will find a way through, around, or over them. It's a sense of calm in your life, no drama, no highs or lows. Your life feels stable and full of promise. I believe that in the midst of madness you can harbor this calm centre, unwavering and you will hear within, the next step to take. A door will always open if you are willing to take that step forward.

Humans have a tendency to put up barriers that not only prevent change from occurring in their lives but also prohibits happiness. A few examples of these doors would be blaming others, feeling ashamed, feeling like a victim, anger, grief, etc., the list is long. There are times in our lives when appropriate and necessary stages of mourning and anger are healthy and essential to process and experience. Getting stuck in any of these emotions, however, is where your life goes off track. Negative and Positive thoughts cannot coexist in the mind. Make a choice.

Step 1: DEFINE HAPPINESS FOR YOU!

Be honest with yourself and assess your happiness on a scale of one to ten. Do you feel any sense of happy, a great sense of happy, or wonder what happy even means? Considering our long history when man focused on survival, the pursuit of happiness was not an affordable luxury. Now consider how recently our technology-assisted lives have changed. Research is finding that in the past, the desire for happiness was actually considered a weakness or not considered at all. Instead, we focused mostly on money, marriage, career, competition and children. Success in many of these areas was often measured by numbers and highlighted by the impermanence of happiness.

Research has found that around 80% of North Americans today report that they are happy. Examining the findings more closely however, shows peoples' lives inundated with flashes of happiness and temporary states of well-being but that it is rare that the state of happiness is actually understood by people.

Keep in mind that we are a culture that values risk, excitement and danger which put these attributes in a positive category for the self. While balance, moderation and happiness are considered dull by our society, these three characteristics are the very foundation from which we can appreciate and safely choose excitement and risk. We forget that we are supported by the universe, and we all have within us that powerful force that sustains all life.

Happy people have younger hearts, younger arteries, and are younger in mind and body than other people the same age. Happy people recover more quickly from trauma, cope better with pain, have lower blood pressure, and have longer life expectancy than unhappy people. Studies show that happy people may have stronger immune systems, are less likely to get colds and flu viruses and, when they do; their symptoms tend to be mild.

Happy and smiling, often go hand in hand. A smile releases endorphins, those happiness signals that surge through our bodies and brains and convince our inner selves that we are happy, confident and satisfied. When we direct a genuine smile at another person, we feel a noticeable sense of happiness.

The physiology of Happiness is important to understand. The brain produces more than fifty identified chemicals. There are over twenty different endorphins alone; some are the brain's painkillers, which are three times more potent than morphine. The release of endorphins has been shown to increase happiness, assist people to push through pain, decrease hunger, and increase the immune response. Scientific research over the last several decades has led to the revolutionary discovery of opiate-like chemicals in the body including serotonin, a hormone manufactured by your brain.

Serotonin is a chemical that helps maintain a "happy feeling" and keeps our moods under control by helping with sleep, calming anxiety, and relieving depression. The brain also makes dopamine, which makes people more talkative and excitable. It affects brain processes that control movement, emotional response, and the ability to experience pleasure and pain. All of these chemicals are natural and affect our bodily processes. A diet deficient in omega-3 fatty acids (sources include flax seeds and fish oils) may lower brain levels of serotonin and cause depression. Managing serotonin levels in your body can be supported by attention to the little things that make you feel good and intentionally include them in your daily routine. Endorphins affect happiness. Their release causes the sensation of feeling good. When our dopamine system is activated, we are more positive, excited and eager to go after goals or rewards. All the brain chemicals you produce are part of a closed loop. They also affect our thinking so that what we focus on expands. If you hold on to happiness it becomes the favored path of your brain, and will not only maintain a level of happiness but will increase that level of happiness. The same of course is true of worry and fear, which lead the brain to produce cortisol, the stress hormone. The stress path the brain follows becomes a habit that is difficult to break, whereas the happy path the brain follows opens doors to many possibilities and opportunities.

Happiness has been linked to increased activity in the brain's left prefrontal lobe, as well as a decreased amount of the stress hormone cortisol in the bloodstream. Cortisol negatively impacts the immune system. With a reduction of T cell function, stressed people have a reduced ability to fight infection and disease. Negative emotions can intensify a variety of health threats and distress-related immune problems. Therefore the opposite is true: staying calm, being optimistic, expressing your feelings and having close personal relationships are all good ways to boost your immune system and help you maintain your health. As Bob Marley sings, 'Don't worry, Be Happy!' Even if you are a recluse and consider yourself friendless, begin with building a close relationship with yourself and you will find you can then reach out to another.

Scientists recognize the role of dopamine in controlling mood as well. Laughing produces endorphins, and when we're happy, we're less stressed, so we don't produce as much cortisol with its damaging effect on our bodies and minds.

Being your own best friend is critical to your success. You might know your best friend's, your spouse's or your child's triggers for happiness better than your own. **Begin a list of what makes you happy, on both a minute scale and the grand scheme of things**. Be honest with yourself in this regard. It is important to differentiate between what we think makes us happy, and what intuitively makes us happy in relationship to our overall goals in life. An example of this would be money and the things we want. Most people think that money would or could make them happy. Go deeper into your life vision; consider all the values that make up your version of joy and success in your life. Once all the thinking is done bring it through the heart and then you will hear the truth of what will make you happy. Fit these into your life plan and your daily activities whenever possible. The rewards are obvious; when we do what makes us happy, what makes us feel good, we support the happiness feedback loop that the brain is designed to create and manage for us.

Step 2: MAKE THE DECISION!

Most people spend approximately eight hours sleeping and eight hours working. What do you do with the other eight hours? Remember, we get to choose not only our actions but our reactions and observations and how they affect our next step, our next choice. The most important person in your life is You. From that simple decision, that you have value, that you have potential and untapped talent and wisdom, arises optimism and the impetus to move forward. You have every right to be optimistic. Optimism is a mental attitude that interprets situations and events as being best. The more broad concept of optimism is the understanding that all of nature, past, present and future, operates by laws of optimization. Being optimistic, in the typical sense of the word, ultimately means one expects the best possible outcome from any given situation. Become aware of your thoughts. Choose your thoughts carefully because, as Mahatma Gandhi said:

"Your beliefs become your thoughts,
Your thoughts become your words,
Your words become your actions,
Your actions become your habits,
Your habits become your values,

Your values become your destiny."

Stress is the cause of most disease whether it took root decades ago or more recently. Stress is your body's response to situations that require a physical, mental or emotional response. It is important for you to understand healthy and useful stress which can elevate you to surpass your expectations and get an A+ on an exam, rescue someone in need or find that answer within that you didn't know you could. Similar to the stress on a material that can no longer bear the weight of an object, your body, mind, heart and soul continually works overtime to support your life in the face of negative stress. How would you measure your daily routine stress levels, both positive and negative? Routine daily stress impairs the prefrontal cortex, the part of the brain responsible for decision making, correcting errors and assessing situations. Our society has become so tolerant of stress, that we have replaced contentment with an acceptable level of stress that we have learned to cope with, which of course has led us to forget what happiness really means in our lives.

We have forgotten not only who we are, but what we are. While people struggle and stress over what to be when they finally grow up, or how to fit into a society that offers them little, we forget why we are here. We have forgotten why our life itself has enormous and awesome value. We have become a people that have to see it to believe it. Yet what we can't measure or see, what most of us never suspect exists, is the silent but irresistible power that comes to the rescue for those who fight on in the face of discouragement. Your body is an organism that is not only a walking miracle, but a complex arrangement of many systems all working together through Body Intelligence; trillions of cells communicating and responding to deliver for your pleasure and performance an awesome life. You get to choose, you get to be the director and star in your own life.

Most of us are familiar with the Serenity Prayer. Here is the original first paragraph of the poem written by Dr. Reinhold Niebuhr in 1932. *"God, give us grace to accept with serenity the things that cannot be changed, Courage to change the things which should be changed, and the Wisdom to distinguish the one from the other."* This small prayer alone can help you move forward, make decisions, and find a way to solve the impossible in any area of your life.

No matter how noisy and fearsome your life may be at this moment, you can learn to listen to the source of wisdom within yourself anytime you want. You don't have to look around for confirmation from anyone else, or even consider how they think you should choose or respond. You don't have to consult memories of how you behaved dozens of times in similar situations. You simply tap into your own inner voice and direction will come. Believe in yourself, stop underestimating the limitless possibilities and your ability to tap into 'life' itself to prosper, thrive and be happy. Stop using words like I can't, I won't, it's impossible, or I am afraid. Begin your sentence with I may, I will, yes I can, I have nothing to fear, and give your brain permission to find a way.

Change your mental attitude and the world around you will change accordingly. **You create your own reality, with each decision you make, each thought you think. Learn to control your thoughts; don't let your thoughts control you.** Don't settle for less than the best for yourself. What is in your true best interest is also in the best interest of the world around you, the people you love and the people that count on you. It's where success begins. It's the opposite of the age old 'everyone else comes first' mindset. Consider that most people want the same things: safety, nourishment and love. What is truly best for you means that, if you pursue it whole-heartedly, it is also in the best interest of those around you. When you choose a positive course you set in motion an unstoppable force that will allow you to change your world.

Step 3: BE GRATEFUL!

The solutions we seek for physical health, happiness, success and joy, all rest in ones' ability to simplify whatever situation confronts us. Break it down, take a step back and assess what's really going on, leave drama and emotion behind, take a breath, and find the truth. You can always find something to be grateful for, no matter how you measure your level of wealth, love or joy in your life. For starters, if you are reading this, your heart must be beating! Be grateful. You are already a walking miracle. Be grateful!

No matter your situation, take a moment of time to find something or someone in your life to be grateful for. Start each day with gratitude, not hokey melodrama; I am talking of simple, quiet gratitude for your life. **Make a list, put it on the bathroom mirror, begin and end each day with gratitude.** This simplest of steps will change your life. As gratitude replaces complaining and focusing on what is missing, your life will begin to fill with good.

Religions are man's many different interpretations of the spiritual realm. There are as many names for God as there are cultures and languages from the past to the present time. When we speak of Greater Intelligence, the source of all that is, all that is greater than what we now know; you want to determine where this spiritual view fits into your life. All that matters is your personal relationship with the divine. Make it right for you.

It matters not what your religious views are, whether or not you believe in one of the many images of God and/or Supernatural Power that is considered the source of all. The word 'believe' is defined as 'to accept as true or real'. What matters is that you recognize (or at least consider) that which is greater than you. It doesn't matter how you phrase it; it matters that you step out of the 'man is the top of the food chain' view and investigate for yourself that there is a greater intelligence than you; that this universe, this life, this breath you take comes from a source unseen. With this critical acknowledgement you elevate your life. Be Grateful!

The systematic study of gratitude within psychology only began around the year 2000. I am sure this is because psychology has traditionally been focused more on understanding distress rather than understanding positive emotions. Gratitude has become a mainstream focus of psychological research. This research has focused on understanding the short term experience of the emotion of gratitude, individual differences in how often people feel gratitude, and the relationship between these two.

Science now shows that grateful people are happier, less depressed, less stressed, and more satisfied with their lives and social relationships. Grateful people also have higher levels of control of their environments, personal growth, purpose in life, and self acceptance. Grateful people have more positive ways of coping with the difficulties they experience in life, being more likely to seek support from other people, reinterpret and grow from the experience, and spend more time planning how to deal with problems. They also have fewer negative coping strategies, being less likely to try to avoid the problem, deny there is a problem, blame themselves, or cope through substance use. Grateful people sleep better, and this seems to be because they have fewer negative and more positive thoughts just before going to sleep.

Gratitude has been said to have one of the strongest links with mental health of any character trait. The longest lasting effects from a number of research projects were due to the writing of "gratitude journals" wherein participants were asked to write down three things they were grateful for every day. These participant's happiness scores continued to increase each time they were periodically tested thereafter. In fact, the greatest benefits were usually found to occur around six months after journaling began. It was so successful that, although participants were only asked to continue the journal for a week, many participants continued to keep the journal going long after the study was over. Similar results have been found from studies conducted by Emmons and McCullough (2003) and Lyubomirsky et al (2005).

The key is to be grateful. It's wonderful that science is now considering the value of age-old teachings. Say please and thank you--both are forms of gratitude. Listen to yourself and give thanks as often as you can. You will see amazing results.

Step 4: YOUR BEAUTIFUL BRAIN!

How your brain and happiness go together! What you think, you become, what you focus on expands.   How you nourish your brain determines your ability to think/solve/choose and thrive. Your brain is your own personal super computer that can give you the correct answer to any question if you give it the right fuel to run on. Your brain is made up of 100 billion nerve cells forming a trillion plus connections called synapses in a dynamic state of adjusting while responding to the world around you.   Deepak Chopra's book "Superbrain" is a rich and easy read to understand what you are made of and how you can get back into the drivers' seat of your own life. There are endless studies that astound the scientists as they reveal the limitless possibilities of the human brain.

Understand that in each moment, on some level, you choose how you feel and respond. If your life has become one long 'habit' then you will choose the feedback loop that has been playing in your brain for much of your life. Body Intelligence is the culmination of trillions of cells in your body communicating and listening to each other on many levels, every second of every day. When you think a thought, the brain sends information to the heart and if the message is excitement or fear it can make the heart beat faster. The brain then sends a message to make the heart slow down because homeostasis (internal equilibrium) must be managed at all times for health and longevity. Obviously, if stress is high over a long period of time no message is sent to calm down the heart.

In the era of early man, thinking was defined by opposition. We needed enemies in order to survive because having enemies forced us to sharpen our skills of self defense and warfare. We all know the consequences of war. Benjamin Franklin said, "There never was a good war or a bad peace." It is long past mans need to find a better way to solve local and global conflict. Modern politics is based on debate, money, greed, power and posturing; all of which pushes people deeper into their own mind sets instead of cooperating and seeking better solutions and plans. There is a huge difference between listening with a closed mind versus listening with an open mind and an honest desire to understand the opinion being expressed by another. Today we must and can override brain patterns that are no longer relevant.

Deepak Chopra calls for a new trend; 'survival of the wisest' not 'survival of the fittest'. Don't bully others and don't let others bully you. Aggressive, outward bullying behavior is always hiding an internal insecurity and fear. This is true in every case of bullying. So don't be fooled any longer by someone trying to control your life or the life of someone else. Bullying plants the seed of a grudge and many people hold onto grudges for decades. One grudge alone can displace you from your own personal power, your own ability to make the right choice.

Keep in mind it takes decades to become a mature adult. We all know people who are 60 or 70 years old and are yet to be mature adults. Start right now to examine where you stand in the role of mature adult. From birth it takes up to 25 years for the body and brain to reach full function and maximum physical growth. Only then can the evolution of wisdom and emotional maturity, essential building blocks for a fulfilled and happy life, begin.

Being 'right' is insignificant compared to being happy. You must stop struggling, arguing and focusing on the problem because the answer never lies there. You must step out of the drama to find the solution. The road to brain wellness begins with awareness. The facts are - you create your own reality and what you focus on expands. Stop using words like 'I can't', 'I won't', 'I don't know how', 'I can never do that', and 'I am afraid to try'. As soon as you think them or say them, they become your reality.

Since **oxygen** is critical to efficient brain function, breathing in a conscious way will greatly enhance your ability to think. If you safely stop where you are and take 3 long, slow deep breaths in and out, you will fill your brain with oxygen and instantly calm down; it works every time. From there your brain can allow the answer, solution, the first step necessary to move in a happy direction to rise above the brain fog. Use this practice when making tough decisions, solving problems and most importantly when you are resolving conflict.

Read the book "Your Body's Many Cries for Water" (see booklist). Cellular dehydration, even when you have no obvious symptoms, sets the stage for cellular stress and illness. Recognizing that your body is 73-78% water, and your brain is 85% water, it is obvious that hydration is essential for proper brain function and for all body systems to do their job efficiently and energetically.

Drink eight 8-ounce glasses of good water (not chlorinated/fluoridated) every day. Prioritize it and, in as little as 7 days, you will feel a difference in energy levels and clarity of mind. Avoid fluoride—it damages the brain's pineal gland. Evidence against fluoride is a great gift that technology and science have given us; oh, wait, they were the ones that put it in our water in the first place. Carry water with you everywhere you go; at home set a timer to remind you to drink water hourly.

You have a mind and you have a brain. Understand the difference. We have become captive of our brain habits and thoughts. "A simple example: a man is undergoing brain surgery and the doctor presses a part of the brain. The patient's arm rises up. When the doctor asks the patient what happened, he says 'My arm moved up'. Then the doctor asks the patient to move his other arm up in the air and asks the same question, 'What happened?' The

patient says 'I moved my arm up in the air."
(Deepak Chopra, Superbrain) This is a simple
way to show you that the brain and the mind are
two different things. Your mind tells your brain
what you want and the brain delivers. The
brain, your super computer, will repeat the most
frequently used pathways to perpetuate what is
familiar. You must control your brain, not be
controlled by it.

The mind only grows stronger when it is active.
The more you exercise and stretch your brain,
the more opportunities and new ideas will
bubble to the surface. Everyone needs ways to
relax. Instead of **wasting** excessive time
watching TV or participating in other escapist
pastimes that put your brain on 'autopilot',
manage that time in more brain-enhancing
ways. Create time and space for reading and
learning.

Make a decision to use your brain in all you do,
actively consider all your skills as you move
through your day, your job and your play. Keep
in mind that wise persons are those who think
twice before speaking once. Everything you do
will be easier and more satisfying.

If you repeat something over and over to yourself, your subconscious mind will eventually begin to accept it as fact. Once this happens your subconscious mind will work overtime to transform the idea into physical reality. Of course, if you are repeating 'I can't' or 'I'm stupid', then you will easily convince yourself and that will manifest in all you do. Turn this around by thinking positive thoughts and use affirmations to persuade your subconscious that you are capable of doing anything you want to do. Keep it up and your subconscious will eventually manifest this new you. Have notes that are visible in your home when you walk by, on the bathroom mirror or the fridge or on the door before you leave the house. Remind yourself of the positive version of yourself and your life as often as possible, especially whenever you begin to doubt yourself. Your brain is brilliant; it will take hold of the thoughts it hears most and move you into positive territory in your life. I have found one of the phrases that people are most reluctant to say to themselves in the mirror is 'I love myself, I love me.'

For centuries meditation has been used around the world to empower the mind and strengthen the brain. Meditation is now considered the best anti-aging tool we have. Science now teaches us that at the end of every chromosome is the protein enzyme telomerase, a repeating DNA sequence. Telomerase protects DNA from aging and meditation has been found to increase the enzyme telomerase. Consider the brilliance of the mind/body connection. It exists and once you tap into this, your abilities, happiness, and success multiply exponentially. After 7 days of spending 20 minutes a day in meditation, in quiet, open minded personal space, your life will change. The key is to apply these new tools to your life.

Step 5: WHO YOU MASTERMIND WITH!

You are fully loaded, with all the talents, gifts and ability you require to find and create happiness in your life. For most people, the scars of life experience and societal limitations have become a long list of disappointments that are the feedback loops your precious brain continues to ride. Patterns of behavior, addictions and sorrow become the routines of our lives. So many people nurture their scars and sorrow, and focus and remember them so often that unconsciously they fully prevent possibilities of escape. Great or small, a negative thought can divert you from your path of success and happiness. This can even start in the womb through actions or thoughts of mother or father, poor nutrition, or the environment. All of us have multiple examples, from birth to now, of diversions from our own truth due to the impact and drama of this society. These magnify and multiply over time, often to the point that we don't even know why we are here or how to find our way back to our rightful path. No matter what your history, no matter who did what to you, who did or did not love you–none of it matters now. Whoever has affected your life, and no doubt there are many, you can choose to let them go. Consider that they too were victims, so why would you think they could have behaved differently?

Ordinary people who do extraordinary things for others are those we later call heroes. When asked why they performed as they did, they often say, "It was nothing; anyone else would have done the same in the circumstances." I interpret this as a way of saying that we all have the capacity for greatness.

Firstly, remember that you are a 'stand alone', fully loaded for a happy life person from conception to the present moment. Taking this complete YOU forward to connect with masterminds in your life, expands all of your horizons. 'Masterminding' may be defined as: "coordination of knowledge and effort in a spirit of harmony, between two or more people, for the attainment of a definite purpose." (Napoleon Hill, Think and Grow Rich). Hill uses ideas from physics to illustrate the synergy that occurs between like-minded individuals. He also warns of the danger to the mastermind group of any single member who thinks negatively. Another key insight from Hill is that knowledge is not power – it is only potential power. He defines power as "...organized knowledge, expressed through intelligent efforts." The mastermind group makes this happen.

The most important mastermind with which you partner is, of course, you. The second most important is the person you choose as a life partner. Once you realize the awesome life potential within you and have learned to accept yourself as a perfect work in progress, imagine what an awe inspiring relationship you will create when you meet a fellow Mastermind!

If you, like most people have not realized nor found a way to be your absolute best, how can you possibly meet the person that matches you? Sure, in the beginning there is a spark, something special that happens and love grows. However, because of generations of gender-role conditioning and no 'Handbook' to guide you, many relationships slowly (or quickly) lose vitality. You expect in the other person what you never even imagined in yourself. A 54 percent divorce rate in North America corroborates this. Most relationships could succeed with grace and ease if; humility replaced pride, generosity replaced greed, patience replaced anger, and so on. The most important decision you make is the person you choose to spend the rest of your life with, because your future and all of your choices and opportunities are affected by the influence and power of another. Choose well!

Assess who you mastermind with. Napoleon Hill wrote a book called "Outwitting the Devil", a brilliant work about masterminding and incorporating the best the universe has to offer you. Analyze your relationships with family, life partners, co-workers, friends, etc. and determine what they contribute and how they assist in elevating you to a pinnacle of happiness and success.

Do not allow yourself to be lulled into complacency by the masses who believe mediocrity is an acceptable alternative. Focus on success, not failure. If you find yourself doubting your next step reach out to a positive person who wants the best for you. If you find yourself alone in your life then find an organization or group that will welcome you and offer assistance. There are many out there today that are inclusive and generous.

It is important to have safeguards in place as you succeed, as you find happiness. Sad though it sounds, when you start to rise to your rightful place, those who are not on the same path may attempt to sabotage you. Hence, be careful with whom you mastermind, even those you have coffee with, jog with, or plan a party with. Every choice and decision you make can be affected by what others think of your choices, even by those who are there to assist you. So you must be alert, aware and conscious of where you are going and who you desire to go with you. Mediocre people may delight in seeing you fail. This is not to say they are not good people, as most people are inherently good. I am saying that unconsciously people may prefer that you stay the same so they are not left in the ditch themselves. Mediocre people will try to keep you on their level. As a result of this I practice the Law of Silence with people who may not have my best interest at heart. Be careful with whom you share your life plans and dreams with. Successful people are optimistic people. You must know what you want, have a plan that is right for you and stick to it.

So the buck stops with you. Choose for yourself and drop the baggage. Remember, blame is worse than useless. It will hold you back. It is so easy to fall deeper and deeper into the dark. Remember also that **what you focus on**

expands. So calm down and know that you can fix your present no matter what the damage. Take one step at a time. Stop spending your time focusing on what's wrong; focus on what you want and it will find its way to you. This works 100 percent of the time. So prioritize 'happy' and it will find its way to you in small doses, big doses, waves of calm and contentment. This is universal law, what goes around comes around, what you give you get. The universe is a circle and there is no way to make it square with exits and doors and options. This is Truth. Choose your friends, lovers and co-workers with conscious care.

I believe we are meant to be happy. The key to happiness, the key to success in any endeavor is to simplify, sort out the facts and the fakes, get to the root of what is necessary to achieve your goal. I realize that there are millions in the world starving and in crisis who would find this book absurd. However, if you are not one of them, it is your job, your responsibility as a human on this planet to be the best you can be.

Step 6: NOW IS THE ONLY TIME AND PLACE YOU EXIST!

We know NOW that what we focus on expands. It's a fact. Hence the failure of most diets: focusing on the number on your scale means you are focusing on what you have to lose rather than what you have to gain in health and happiness. So focus on happiness and it will prove to be the best diet you were ever on.

No matter what problem you need to solve or question you need to answer, do it in the NOW. We have a tendency to carry forward with us the baggage of our failures, wrong choices, and mistakes, because we live in the past instead of the NOW. We can think ourselves out of success by recalling the number of times we failed, the number of times we picked the wrong paint color, brought home the wrong this or that, and so on. Think about preparing a meal–if there are no clean dishes, if the kitchen is a disaster, if the fridge isn't stocked with the ingredients we need, if the power is out, how can we possibly create a nourishing meal? So, once again, calm down, break it down into steps. Do not over think this. Do the dishes, go to the grocery store, clean the kitchen, and call the power company; whatever steps are needed to complete the project, just do them, one at a time. Be in the NOW, exercise your brain. Even if it's a thousand times a day, just keep gently bringing yourself into the present. Right NOW is the only place that you will find your joy. The past holds nothing for you; the future doesn't exist, so be present NOW and take responsibility for your own happiness. After all, responsibility is simply the ability to respond.

Here's a simple exercise to get you into the NOW and through any decision you have to make: **breathe**. Yes, we have actually forgotten how to breathe. **Breathing consciously will bring you into the NOW faster than any other method.** Most people shallow breathe. This is defined as "thoracic breathing, or chest breathing, which is the drawing of minimal breath into the lungs, usually by drawing air into the chest area using the intercostal muscles rather than throughout the lungs via the diaphragm"(Wikipedia). Oxygen is essential for every cellular activity that takes place in the body. The brain cannot function efficiently without the proper amount of oxygen. Diaphragmatic breathing, abdominal breathing, belly breathing or deep breathing involves slow and deep inhalation through the nose, filling the brain and body with oxygen.

The body has a physiological response to the breath. As the breath is regulated, chemicals in the brain become more balanced; the level of oxygen in cells increases and the heartbeat can slow down. Many people spend a huge amount of time stuck in the 'fight or flight' mechanism that served us well running from a tiger thousands of years ago. That continual level of hyper-awareness and stress exhausts the adrenal glands and eventually we become paralyzed by stress, unable to save our own lives.

Conscious breathing can slow down the mind. By making conscious breathing a habit, the brain begins a new pattern of behavior. Calm becomes the foundation from which we begin to make decisions and react to our lives. According to Ujjayi breathing in Yoga, "The quality of your breath is directly related to your state of mind, so when you are aware of your breath you can be aware of your inner state." (Yogajournal.com) Conscious breathing is a focus on the breath, a perfect way to be in the NOW.

Use a heart-centered breathing practice that will assist you in changing your life. The aim is your full attention and awareness on your breath. Use this slow, deep breath to assist you when solving a problem, answering a difficult question or to calm you in an emotional situation. Slow down your breath, twice daily, for three minutes each time. Inhale to the count of 10, exhale to the count of ten. This is an easy exercise to incorporate into any busy life. The rewards are limitless. You will have revived your brain, raised the quality of your life to where health, happiness, & wealth are possible. Follow this practice for 7 days and you will change your life.

Step 7: BODY INTELLIGENCE!

Every one of your unique trillions of cells is part of a body intelligence that is unmatched in the universe. Think about it. You have a heart, your heart beats. Have you congratulated yourself lately because the body intelligence you possess is designed to heal itself, repair damage and perform the best it can with what you give it? The innate healing system within your body is involuntary. You don't have to think to heal a cut; the body is designed to specifically deal with whatever you come into contact with, provided you give it the correct building blocks with which to work. Many of us had great parents, but perhaps correct nourishment in-utero was missing. Some of us had the worst possible parents, leaving us with serious problems to work out on our own. Take heart, though, because no matter the effect, the damage, the issues, you can fix it now.

Take an interest in your body. We are very specific about what fuel we put into our car, yet we take our body for granted. The connection between our thoughts and our body responses is extremely sensitive; if we are unaware, we can quickly spiral downward into discomfort and disease. And, though doctors put people in crisis back together brilliantly, their success is not great when dealing with chronic or degenerative disease. There is no doubt that a diagnosis can be critical to your decision-making and choice of path toward healing. Use your brilliant brain to investigate and understand the biology of your particular situation and be in charge of your own healing. You choose what's best for you.

The books on diets, performance and beauty abound; yet our population is sicker than ever. Consider the fact that disease can only thrive in an acidic environment—it cannot live in an alkaline environment. Yet the majority of people in the developed world have an acidic environment in their bodies that encourages disease, discomfort and mental illness. Yes, genetic disease also may play a role but one of the greatest gifts you can give yourself is to assess how you have nourished your body up to now. I can tell you this: if you change your body's acidic environment to an alkaline one, all good things will follow.

The correlation between Body Intelligence and food is a fine balance that defines your performance in all areas of your life. You are what you eat is true in every sense of the word.

Try a 7 day organic vegetable/fruit juice diet and you will feel alive again. A positive change in your overall well being in just 7 days will occur. Talk to your doctor if you must; however, it is common sense to fill your body with organic, highly nutritious food. A week is a short time to give yourself a break. Your taste buds, so abused over time, will rejoice to remember the delicious flavor of simple fruits and vegetables. We are so naïve to accept the diet of the day. The masses are overeating while the rest of the world goes hungry.

The cells of your body are replicating and replacing themselves on a continual basis. Cells can only replicate the state they are currently in. If your body has an acidic internal environment, which is conducive to disease, then you recreate this state over and over as your cells divide and replicate themselves. Once you take better care of your body you begin the process of rebuilding yourself with healthy cells.

Our bodies are organic, sacred temples full of bountiful opportunities to enjoy, thrive, dance, sing, and understand simple joy. Assess your daily diet over a 7-day period and decide on one week of change to experience the difference. Become your own experiment and switch to a diet of organic fruits and vegetables. You will not only lengthen your life, but you also begin the process of eliminating disease and discovering vitality and energy. A 7-day organic vegetable/fruit juicing program is not only delicious. It will deliver in a week, a feeling of energy and vitality that you have likely forgotten is possible. You will also lose unnecessary weight with this eating regime. Go ahead and check with your health care practitioner first, listen to their suggestions/ideas/recommendations with your **super brain,** and decide for yourself if this is in your best interest. Don't be foolish enough to think that you must eat meat every day, drink cow's milk every day, you must this or you must that. Think about what your energy output is each day? That will be the key to what you need to consume. Your body needs a break from the routine of inadequate nutrition and a juice fast will thrill your cells. You can drink these delicious drinks all day long. If you don't have a juicer, eat the fruits and veggies whole.

Our bodies are the only vehicle we have in which to experience life. The devastation of 'dis'ease and the costly and painful repair should be incentive enough to take care of your body, mind, heart and soul. We have not evolved long since our hunter/gatherer ancestors. Our bodies are meant to move, to simply walk every day or to take on a sport of our very own. So consider what you have done to your body for years. But don't be hard on yourself; there are a multitude of reasons for your past choices that don't matter anymore. Choose to take action NOW. Any increase in the amount of physical activity in your life will contribute to well-being. Whether it is yoga, biking, weight training, daily walks around the neighborhood, an active sport, or learning wheelchair exercises; move more every day. No more excuses, no more feeling sorry for yourself or tolerating your sad state.

Remember disease cannot live in an alkaline environment. Disease must have an acidic environment in order to prosper. In a nutshell, no matter what your physical ailment might be, the first step is to change the internal environment to alkaline. This alone is a huge leap toward wellness.

Next, eliminate sugar from your diet—another huge leap. Natural sugars in the fruit/vegetables/grains are all you need. We have allowed ourselves to be brainwashed into believing that sugar, preservatives, pesticides, and genetically modified organisms (GMO's) are all contributing to our longevity and quality of life. Realize that TV advertising is a game—someone else's game, designed ONLY to take your money. It is not real life and it has very little to contribute to your best choices for a long, healthy and happy life. So it's time for common sense to take over. Don't make excuses for yourself. Choose differently for as few as 7 days and you'll get the true picture. For too long we have allowed others to decide what we feed our children and ourselves. Get in the habit of reading labels. You don't have to become a rigid food maniac. But I want you to at least investigate balance in your foods. Sugar, meat, dairy, alcohol, smoking all create an acidic internal environment where disease can prosper. If you choose to eat meat a few times a week be sure you are choosing correctly for you both ethically and for your body type. **Balance alkaline foods and hydrate with good water to create good health and healthy thinking.**

Add simple foods that are loaded with nutrition. Give thanks for what you eat. Vegetables, fruits, home grown sprouts, grains (all organic, whenever possible) and good water make cooking simple and highly nutritious. We now know that stress and city living use up your reserves of Vitamin C very quickly. As Vitamin C is water soluble, you eliminate what you don't use on an hourly basis. So consider taking 500 mg Vitamin C with bioflavonoid three times daily to give your body what it needs to resist stress. Including essential fatty acids is critical to a healthy body and mind. Adding organic ground flax seed to meals and taking 1 tbsp. organic flax seed oil daily is a great start.

Chia seeds are a super food. Thirty percent of the Chia seed's oil is Omega 3 and 40% of its oil is Omega 6. Chia Seeds can absorb over ten times their weight in water, making them great for rehydrating our bodies. Include them in your day and fill your body with vitality.

Now is the time. Take an interest and create a sensible plan for yourself. People who are trapped in the societal view of beauty and weight simply have to see themselves as more than a photograph. You are what you eat—it's true. If you are not eating simple, wholesome foods described in this book, you are contributing to your own problems. Take action, especially since these suggestions have no bad side effects. Take a step back to see yourself for the amazing creature you truly are. Above all else, be kind to yourself. You have such value and potential that you owe it to yourself to throw out the image of what you have been and see instead what you can become.

Your body requires correct foods to give you peak performance in mind, body, heart and soul. Yes, the addictions are tough to face, the habits and behaviors perhaps tough to change; but YOU get to decide your fate. Only seven days of good choices will give you results that will inspire you and get you through the next seven days. This program follows the long-held understanding of the cycles of 7 that are at work in our lives. Each successful 7 days of change gets your brain's attention. "She/he must be serious this time." Each 7 days you shift bad habits to good. Every experience you have turns into a message that can alter the health and life of your individual cells. It really is that easy!

Step 8: RECONNECT WITH NATURE!

Remember that the universe and all that is in it are made from tiny atoms, as is your body and your internal universe. The universe is a closed system; there are no additions or deletions from the physical world we know. You are part of the world you live in. On average today, a person in contemporary society lives 90% of his or her life devoid of conscious sensory contact with nature. Many spend over 90% of their time indoors. We think, write and build relationships while closeted from nature. This disconnected state fools us into believing that our extreme separation from nature does not influence our intelligence, sanity or ability to relate responsibly. Unlike nature-connected cultures, our detachment from nature's workings psychologically deprives our thinking of elements that hold life in balance. It is essential to reconnect with nature to know who and what you are. It is the easiest way to rekindle a true desire to value and care for yourself properly.

A child advocacy expert, Richard Louv was the first to collect and expose a growing body of evidence suggesting healthy physical, emotional and mental development in both children and adults requires direct interaction with nature. In his latest book, "The Nature Principle," Louv suggests humanity's reliance on technology has subverted our connection with nature. We have hamstrung our ability to know the universe more fully via direct knowledge of the essence of nature. It goes without saying our ability to enhance our lives through the power of nature has been reduced. We must pay attention to the restorative powers of the natural world, which science has shown can improve mental acuity, creativity, health and wellness, our concepts of sustainability, families and communities, businesses and economies and, most important of all, our connections with each other and all beings.

A mere decade ago man lived closer to nature. With ever-growing populations living in cities we have become not only sedentary but computerized and televised and out of touch. The paradox of the term 'concrete jungle' is perfect. Imagine the ease of standing in a peaceful forest, the sound of birds, feeling the breeze on your face and compare that to standing in a downtown big city surrounded by concrete, electromagnetic radiation and the ever-present sounds and smells of traffic, construction, congestion, etc.

You can, however, begin the reconnecting process by simply growing plants in your home, connecting with trees in the park or on your street in the city, taking a few moments to silently appreciate the sky and the birds, or taking a walk in the woods. Listening instead of talking, re-creating a relationship with silence (not filling your ears and eyes with TV/computers/music/noise)…just for a change, just for moments each day. No matter where you are, look around and see the beauty. You may have to look far and deep in some places to see beauty, but if you do you will be totally present, focused in the moment you are living.

In 1989 two whales were trapped in the arctic winter ice and became international superstars. To save the whales, opposing nations united, bridging the hostility between communism and capitalism. So too did labor and industry, corporations and environmentalists, spiritualists and scientists, technologists, peacemakers and the media. Close to a billion dollars was spent to save two whales by cutting them a path through the arctic ice to freedom while the world cheered and unified.

This experience demonstrated that the attractions we feel when in contact with a whale or other form of nature are but the tip of an iceberg (pun intended). Like whales, we humans are part of nature and we have forgotten that our true goals are peace and celebration. Reconnecting with nature is about re-awakening ourselves to who we really are and discovering the true nature of our existence.

Our industrialized and technological societies have separated us from the Earth and from each other. Too many children now think food comes from cans and boxes. Too many adults believe the meaning of life is about paying a mortgage and buying bigger and better stuff.

All lives on the planet, all the plants and creatures, including us, are in this together. We have the instinct, ability and responsibility to get along. A moose is so good at being a moose, living and thriving throughout long winters merely on the growing tips of trees. We humans have forgotten how to be human and be part of the great plan of nature on our planet. When we reconnect to nature, we start to see the world the way we were meant to see it; we are integral to it, not separate from it. Nature is part of the foundation of all communities, and essential to your reconnection to the earth that feeds and houses you.

Just a few steps will get you there; get outside, eat nature's food, learn to sit still, live mindfully and be alert to your senses. Pay attention, and make good choices.

Step 9: SAVE YOUR OWN LIFE!

Absolutely no one else can do this for you. If you are a woman, you have been taught for millennia that everyone else comes first. If you are a man, you have never been taught how to care for yourself on levels that matter.

The greatest gift we have to offer each other is the work we do on ourselves. You have experienced being in the presence of a person who is happy, exudes confidence, smiles a lot and shows grace and caring. It is a contagious feeling and for those moments you are lifted up as well. That is how powerful a smile, a positive approach and a determined happy person contributes to a better world. Likewise, negativity and greed are also infectious and contagious. They can kill, destroy, maim, steal, and limit not only your present, but also your future. Both are powerful; pay attention, make good choices.

Opportunity comes in many disguises. Thomas Edison's failures were not failures, but simply opportunities to rule out what didn't work. If you manage your emotions and maintain a critical eye to what needs to change, success will follow. Napoleon Hill, in his book 'Shake

Hands with The Devil' speaks of the gold miner who quit three feet from the mother lode. What a perfect analogy for not stopping short of success. If everything we attempted in life was achieved with a minimum of effort and came out exactly as planned, how little we would learn and how boring life would be! Failure is always one of life's great learning experiences. You can be absolutely certain that when you feel you are being most unfairly tested, you are actually preparing for great success.

Your view of yourself greatly influences how others perceive you. If you are a confident, cheerful, positive person, your co-workers, friends, and family will be drawn to your personality. If you are unhappy, negative, and always complaining about your situation, people will avoid being near you. The old saying, *'fake it till you make it,'* is a simplification of Aristotle's notion that acting virtuous will make one virtuous. Putting 'fake it till you make it' into action in your life will work every time as you move forward to find the truth and joy within you. You will find that you soon feel genuinely more positive, because your subconscious mind believes you and has faith in you no matter what. Only you can save your own life, and only you can define what that looks like.

Actively seek to be an enlightened person. In original Sanskrit 'enlightenment' means liberation. It is easy to see the big picture and observe the universe and recognize brilliance at work, the perfect plan that created this place. Once you accept that you are part of everything, your entire life view will change. Have an open mind about spirituality. Welcome divine presence in your life; however you define it. Remember that what you resist; persists. To override worry you have to create the awareness that the actual fear doesn't exist. Not to disregard physical safety and some crisis people find themselves in. That is a different matter and requires action. However, much of what we fear doesn't really exist. As in days gone by when running from tigers may have been part of our reality, today most of what we fear is in our own minds. If you focus on solutions, regardless of the complexity, you will bring measureable security and confidence into every aspect of your life.

Deepak Chopra suggests mindfulness is a state of creative potential and self-awareness. Take the challenge and experience it for 20 minutes daily by breathing deeply in a calm and quiet place. A few examples from a very long list include enhanced immune system, decreased aging, increased emotional stability and a renewed feeling of peace and happiness. Do the research yourself and decide to give yourself this gift.

Make peace with yourself and your situation. From there, infuse your thoughts and actions with awareness and consciousness and you begin to see that you *are* the world. You are not *in* the world, the world is *in* you. Why else are you here other than to be the best you can possibly be? You are endowed with unique gifts and talents. You have an awesome life worth saving. Begin today to live it to the fullest.

Step 10: STOP BEING NAÏVE!

Making assumptions about anyone or any situation is naïve. Assuming people are who they say they are is naïve. It is very positive and optimistic to look for the truth in people, places and experiences you have. However it is only when *you* come from a place of truth, that you will know what is right for you or wrong for you. If most of the people around you are guessing at success, negative about their lives and not aware that they are missing happiness, can they have answers for *your* life? No one can do more for you than they can do for themselves. Television, news media, governments, & even schools are all part of this 'unhappy' mess. You must become discerning and make right choices for yourself. Simplify information as it comes to you. Don't take it as fact. Don't adopt it without serious consideration. Just as you may sometimes be your own worst enemy, unconsciously choosing badly, you can also be your own best friend. The switch usually occurs when you realize that the only person on earth who can determine your failure or success is you.

If you have the courage that comes from the sincere conviction that you are an honest, dependable, kind, and caring person, you will never have to worry about what others think of you. The only limits you have in mind, body and heart are limits you impose on yourself. If you are a procrastinator you are wasting time and sabotaging your success on every level. Stop explaining and start doing! Control your own mind and you will never be controlled by other people, government, or any form of media.

When you make the decision to become a person of integrity, you will also find that you are willing to do the right thing simply because it is the right thing to do.

In moments of conflict, your voice can easily betray your anger, fear, or despair instead of the wisdom you could offer. Your tone alone can erase your best message. Listen to yourself, stick to your principles, and you will know that you have protected the most important thing you have, your true self. Know that in the worst of calamities and the toughest of tragedies, staying calm and alert will serve you better than any kind of emotional response.

It is an interesting part of human nature that some people see opportunities, while others only see problems. Know yourself and don't be naïve about who you are and know that all things are possible for you. **Realistically assess your strengths and weaknesses.** Identify what areas you are best in and those where you need improvement. Work on your weaknesses and build upon your strengths so that when you recognize opportunities you will know how to incorporate them into your life. Add to your skill set, diversify your interests and have fun with learning new things on a regular basis.

Step 11: DEFINE YOUR PURPOSE!

Figure out your purpose – everything else is easy.

Skeptics have the opinion that they have to see it to believe it. The Truth is you have to **believe it in order to see it.** The physical body you inhabit, no matter what complicated view you may have, is a collection of atoms vibrating at enormous speed, all working together to create *you*. The source of life is to be honored, respected and appreciated. A miracle is defined as an effect or extraordinary event in the physical world that surpasses all known human or natural powers. As such, life itself qualifies as a miracle. So celebrate that you are here, with limitless potential to manifest a super life for yourself.

Far too many people spend their lives waiting for that glorious day when *the* perfect opportunity presents itself to them. Look instead to each day for small *or* great opportunities. You will begin to notice that, if you are in a state of readiness to receive, opportunities will find you. **Formulate a plan** for everything you would like to accomplish in your life, however large or small.

The imagination is the workshop of your life. This is where you take copious notes and infuse your mind with optimism and grace as you formulate your plans for achievement. Your mind is not constrained by physical limitations or boundaries. It is said that Albert Einstein visualized how the universe might look if he were riding astride a beam of light through infinity. Then he worked out the mathematics to support his theory of relativity. You can use the power of your imagination to visualize solutions to difficult problems, to develop new ideas, and to see yourself achieving the goals you have set for yourself.

Most obstacles in life will succumb to consistent, sustained, intelligent, positive action. Thomas Edison 'failed' thousands of times before perfecting the incandescent electric light bulb. He had an extraordinarily positive perception of life that greatly enhanced his abilities as an inventor. He quite simply viewed each unsuccessful experiment as the elimination of a solution that wouldn't work, thereby moving him that much closer to a successful solution. **Nurture curiosity in your life.** Children love to seek answers and explore and wonder why. If you recapture even a small part of the curiosity you had as a child, your view of your life would explode into possibilities. When you believe in your ideas and your abilities, and you trust in the Infinite Intelligence of the universe, you cannot fail.

Time and again we hear stories about ordinary people who perform Herculean feats of strength and endurance, things they never dreamed they were capable of doing. Imagine harnessing that strength and making it available to your task at hand. Where does that uncanny, super strength go when the heroic event has passed? Finding this super resource within is possible through our inner intelligence. You can, if you believe you can. Success occurs when you have a purpose for your life and you follow through with action. Your goals don't have to be earth-shaking. Your purpose can simply be *happiness*; from there all good things will come to you.

If you focus on trivial matters, blame, shame and self pity, your achievements will be unimportant. Small minds think about small things. **Great minds think about ideas and opportunity.** Discipline yourself to think about what is in your best interest. Flip the switch to focusing on what is best for you, what makes you happy, what is essential for your shift to positive thinking. Take the next step with optimism and a positive attitude. It will expand.

Abraham Lincoln once observed, "You can fool some of the people all of the time, and all of the people some of the time, but you cannot fool all of the people all of the time." Confidence and self-respect carry undeniable weight and will set you apart from the pretenders in all situations. If you discover you are a pretender, then likely you are unnoticed by those who might offer you opportunity. People will take notice in your life when you become your true self. You must treat others with respect, and you will begin to draw good relationships to you. The universe is characterized by order and harmony. Apply this in your life and your purpose will become your reality.

Avoid worry at all cost. Do **what** you can **when** you can in your present situation. Don't play the 'what if' game, unless you are focusing on solutions. Worry is absolutely unnecessary and useless at all times. If you send your children out into the world, send them out with angels and prayers and light and let them go. On some level worry is at the root of all stress and will actually sabotage good intentions.

Throw it out; replace it with confidence and trust. Take action, know what you want and make a plan—unless a life of mediocrity is okay with you. We each choose our destiny. Make sure you establish standards for yourself that exceed societal minimums, including the language you use. Mark Twain once observed that 'the difference between the right word and the almost right word is the difference between lightning and a lightning bug." Profanity is simply a sign of inadequate vocabulary and most likely unsound judgment.

If you don't believe in yourself, don't ask anyone else to. People far too easily express their doubts and insecurities to others through body language, tone of voice, inflection, word choice, and other subtle actions. **Make a list of all the things you like about yourself and the things you would like to change.** Feeling sorry for yourself breeds either pity or contempt from others. Avoid it at all times. You are never helpless. Self pity shares similar characteristics to other addictions. People develop a tolerance for them and require larger and larger doses to achieve the same effect. Self pity can become a habit, one so debilitating that you will rob yourself of all the potential you possess. **"We** are what we repeatedly do. **Excellence, then, is not an act, but a habit.**" (Aristotle, 384 BC – 322 BC)   So don't waste your precious time comparing yourself to others.

Step 12: SMILE AND HEAR MUSIC!

There are so many reasons to smile. Look around as you move through your day and see how many people are not smiling. A smile can be as subtle as a twinkle in the eyes or a broad smile of the mouth. Psychologists have found that even if you are in a bad mood, you can instantly lift your spirits by forcing yourself to smile. 'Fake it till you make it' yet again. Your body is more relaxed when you smile, which contributes to good health and a stronger immune system. In a study conducted in Sweden, people had difficulty frowning when they looked at other subjects who were smiling, and their muscles twitched into smiles all on their own. Your body releases endorphins when you smile, even when you force it. Your body has to work harder and use more muscles to frown than it does to smile. Smiling is a universal sign of happiness. Babies are born with the ability to smile. Smiling makes a person more attractive, sociable and confident, and people who smile more are more likely to get a promotion. People can recognize smiles from up to 300 feet away, making it the most easily recognizable facial expression. A study conducted by Orbit Complete discovered that

69% of people find women more attractive when they smile than when they are wearing makeup.

Watch this validation video to get the total picture of the power of a smile. http://www.youtube.com/watch?v=Cbk980jV7Ao&feature=share

Choose to smile at every opportunity, and welcome music in your life. Music is an essential part of every culture on the planet. Music can calm nerves and soothe emotions. Health benefits in adults who listen regularly to music include slowing down the onset of Alzheimer's disease, lowering blood pressure, and relieving stress. The study of music helps fight depression and mental disorders in adults. Music affords adults the opportunity to explore their creative side and release frustrations. Most people have an automatic emotional response to a favorite song. Playing an instrument and listening to music also provide social opportunities. Music helps with job skills such as creative thinking, collaboration, expressive communication, and confidence. Music helps the process of thinking and learning. Neurological evidence proves that listening to Mozart can raise your IQ. Focusing on music can also prolong attention span and encode information in memory and improve its recall. When you need to do your best brainwork, music can prime and sharpen your mind. Because music is processed on both sides of the brain, listening to it primes your mind to be both artist and scientist, intuitive and logical. Music can coordinate right-brain imagery with left-brain analysis to help you solve problems more creatively, generate imagery to remove creative blocks, and expand your perceptual horizons.

Intentionally smile at every opportunity and create access to your favorite music.

Step 13: HEALTHY RELATIONSHIPS!

Ten thousand plus years of oppositional roles for males and females continues to sabotage the possibility of long lasting love and joy between any two people. It is my understanding that the differences that matter between men and women are simply biological. Again we have been so sculpted by history and our different societies that we have surrendered to the roles imposed upon us. As I stated previously, the greatest gift we can offer another is the work we do on ourselves.   Because we enter into most relationships with a societal view of how that relationship should progress and develop, we initiate a path of struggle and most likely, collapse. Most long term relationships begin with love and joy and celebration and very quickly become peppered with stress and misunderstanding.   If children present themselves quickly in a relationship then the divide is even greater as the children consume all the attention and time of primarily the mother, though there is a new generation of both parents sharing the tasks of raising young.

Here's how it could go – know and love yourself; be prepared to meet in the middle of any and all issues that arise and communicate with truth and respect; keep love as a focus no matter the financial, job, or pressures that you face; listen more than you speak and always tell the truth. Fundamentally all the same truths apply whether in friendship, business, romance, financial or any other relationships that require attention and tending. Starting out with the truth is easier than fixing what you may have had ongoing for years, even a few years set with a backdrop of stress and or old-thinking will require effort to shift to a trusting, respecting and helping relationship foundation. I advise all young people I can to establish that solid and loving relationship with the self, ironed out with truth and great listening skills before ever venturing down the path of creating a long term love affair with another. Don't mistake speaking the truth always with dragging forward all your experiences of the past. This may be factual information, but not always helpful or necessary as you build a solid foundation in a relationship with another. I am not suggesting withholding critical information, I am simply saying live in the moment.

After all, love is why we are here.

Taking a step back, knowing ourselves, knowing what we can give and what we want of any other people who are intimately in our lives, are a few of the steps to make sense of any relationship. At the very least if we were to hire an employee, create a business partnership, share our toys, give of our generosity and trust to anyone, we must wisely have a clear understanding of what is best for us and the other, in order to be 'care' full with our hearts, future, finances and fun. The simplicity of a successful relationship is stunning actually.

What do you want? What do they want? How can you meet each other's needs with grace, happiness and find success? Of course it all points to our ability to know ourselves and have the communication skills to most importantly listen and secondly speak the truth as we know it.

What gets in the way is thousands of years of programming and role playing. What worked then doesn't work now.

Most of us have observed how it appears that time flies, how quickly the years seem to go by from when we were young and full of inspiration to now, when we might wonder where it all went. Love and success can be constructed or reconstructed at any age. Romance at any time can come alive, with truth and intention and willingness to be open. Not understanding the opposite sex is no different than not understanding the same sex if a love relationship is the question. Don't accept the premise, the age old view that men and women are from some opposing force or planet. Read 'The Gate to Women's Country' (see booklist) to get a grasp of what is possible. No matter your sexual orientation, this book will enlighten you. In any relationship two people can create a whole that is greater than the sum of its parts. If the person you are with doesn't believe it is possible, then move on to someone who is willing to see beyond the stereotype and simply be in communion with another human being and prosper and thrive in love.

I do not want to suggest that separation and divorce are simple matters. The fact is we made choices that have led to the NOW in our lives and setting the fear and the drama aside is our only option to survive and move forward in the correct direction for us. When children are involved the fear and difficulty multiplies immensely, however what is best for each of us is always best for those we love the most. Ask for help, plan each step of the way, tell your children the Truth, and not your version of the truth. I am speaking of **The Truth** and find the strength to stand solidly in what is right and just for the life you are living, and for the life of your children. For many people in unfulfilling relationships, the choices and actions to make it right are more obvious. If a partner is unwilling to listen; to want to move forward; to change; or unwilling to understand your request then take the next step. It is my belief that most people want to thrive. The task at hand is to find a wondrous way to demonstrate love, to discuss love, to have enthusiasm and faith that you can succeed in love and reflect it to your partner. Great leadership occurs not as a result of demands; a great leader is defined by example and action, not words.

I love to mentor couples asking the tough questions, insisting on the tough, honest answers. Time is of the essence and not a moment need be wasted in anger and frustration or rebellion and demands. **Stop, listen, and then listen some more** and offer up what you want. Most of us truly want the same thing. Compassion, trust, fun, companionship, love in all its glorious forms, and an open line of communication to speak our hearts and our minds and be heard. How ludicrous it is to be 'married', 'in love' or bound to anyone for any reason and not be able to honestly speak our heart's desire. It is ridiculous to even entertain the thought that marriage/love/commitment could be held together by anything other than the truth between two people. I am not speaking of the truth of the past, or the future, most definitely not the drama of what so many of us have orchestrated in our lives and our relationships. I am speaking of the truth of the now, what we want, what we hope for, what we believe to be possible in our lives and most importantly what we deserve.

'Get real' is such a good instructive action. Why mess with the drama of falsehood. If we don't want to be with someone, don't be with him/her. If we want to build a life together for a day, a month, a lifetime, speak it and lay it out with compassion and truth. There is one issue that, in varying degrees infiltrates many people's lives and often prevents them from choosing the correct action. That issue is guilt.

Vernon Howard (Secrets of Life) addresses the guilt factor very well. Guilt can be a trick you can use to avoid your own responsibilities or a way for others to make you feel guilty over their mistakes. We are not required to sacrifice our lives for others; and mostly guilt reflects an inability to be honest with ourselves and situations. Get Real!

It is your life to live as you choose. You have to do it for yourself. Don't waste time being a victim, living in blame or shame because of whatever. Face up to yourself, care enough about yourself to do what's right for you and those you love. It really is that simple. As Sara Bareilles sings, **'I want to see you be Brave!'**

Checklist

Invest in yourself. From this decision and action you will create opportunities in your life, expand your happiness, improve all of your relationships and move yourself forward step by step to manifesting the awesome and brilliant life you dreamed possible in your youth.

1. **Define Happiness for You**! Begin a list of what makes you happy, on both a minute scale and in the grand scheme of things.
2. **Make a Decision!** Negative and Positive thoughts cannot coexist in the mind. Learn to control your thoughts; don't let your thoughts control you.
3. **Be Grateful!** Make a list, begin and end each day with gratitude.
4. **Your Beautiful Brain!** Respect and care for your beautiful Brain, Hydrate and Breathe Correctly. You are a genius, oh yes you are!
5. **Mastermind with Masterminds!** Choose to mastermind only with people who will elevate you.
6. **Be in the Now!** What you focus on expands. Breathing consciously will

bring you into the now faster than any other method.

7. **Take an interest in your Body!** Go on a 7 day organic vegetable/fruit juice diet and you will feel alive again. Balancing alkaline foods and hydrating with good water equals good health and healthy thinking.

8. **Reconnect with Nature!** You are part of it.

9. **Save your own life!** You deserve it!

10. **Stop being Naïve!** Realistically assess your strengths and weaknesses.

11. **Define your purpose!** Formulate a Plan!

12. **Smile!** Smile at every opportunity.

13. **Healthy Relationships!** Know and speak the truth and the truth shall set you free.

A Few Great Books to Assist You:

Batmanghelidj, F. 2008. Your Body's Many Cries for Water: You're Not Sick; You're Thirsty: Don't Treat Thirst with Medications, 3rd edition, Global Health Solutions.

Chopra, Deepak & Rudolph E. Tanzi. 2012. Superbrain, Harmony Books.

Emoto, Masaru, 2005. The True Power of Water, Beyond Words Publishing Inc.

Hill, Napoleon, 2011. Outwitting the Devil: The Secret to Freedom and Success, The Napoleon Hill Foundation.

Louv, Richard, 2011. *The Nature Principle: Human Restoration and the End of Nature-Deficit Disorder* (Algonquin Books)

Tepper, Sherry S. 1988. The Gate to Women's Country, Bantam Books

Toll, Eckhart, 1997. The Power of Now, Namaste Publishing

Watterson, Bill. 1985-1995 Calvin and Hobbes, Universal Press Syndicate

MY "TO DO" LIST

1. Laugh MORE.
2. Take precise nutritional care of my body each day.
3. Drink more water.
4. Finish book 2 of my 12 book series.
5. Breathe consciously 20min. every day, not every other day.
6. Turn my bad habits into good habits one step at a time.
7. Congratulate myself on progress, big or small.